The Ibogaine Journey

Copyright ©2018 Marco Marcopolis

This book is non-fiction. It is a real-life journey of an opiate addict who made a last-ditch effort to rid himself of a crippling addiction. After desperately trying and failing at every available option in the United States, he traveled to Mexico for Ibogaine treatment. His journey grabs readers into his entire adventure, starting with his research and the difficulties in filtering out the half-truths and misinformation, into his decision making, weighing out the benefits and risks, through his 8-day treatment in Cancun. You'll relive his emotional and physical states, understand what happens during treatment, and what you can expect as an Ibogaine patient. This is a great book for anyone who is thinking about Ibogaine treatment, nervous about the risks, confused about what to believe, and full of questions about the experience. Every page in this book is 100% truthful

The author has dedicated himself to helping others find the right Ibogaine treatment clinics. Please feel free to contact him at findthewaycoach@gmail.com.

Ibogaine Journey:

The Ibogaine Journey is the story of an opiate addict

who decided as a latch ditch effort to try a substance

illegal in the United States to cure him of his addiction.

Relive his journey that led him overseas on an

unforgettable adventure in a quest to leave his

addiction behind him, start a new life without opiates,

and welcome back his former self. The Ibogaine

Journey grabs readers and injects them into the

author's life a few weeks prior to going to Cancun for

Ibogaine treatment, and have them ride though the

research, decision making, and Ibogaine experience.

Learn how this naturally occurring substance found in

the roots of a bush in Africa is astonishing medical

professionals and opiate addicts around the world with

its miraculous properties and abilities to change the

brain chemistry in addicts.

The Ibogaine Journey is an amazing story and a must

read for addicts and loved ones of addicts thinking

about using Ibogaine to treat their addiction. Uncover

the reality of Ibogaine in a sea of mis information and

half-truths.

Is Ibogaine the miracle plant thousands of recovered

opiate addicts claim it to be? Or is it a highly-dangerous

substance that unqualified opportunists administer to

desperate addicts?

You'll finish the Ibogaine Journey having a much better understanding of Ibogaine Treatment, the experience, and the expected outcomes.

Let the author's experience, his advice for finding truthful information about Ibogaine, and your own research lead you to the right decision about whether to use Ibogaine to treat opiate addiction.

The author has dedicated his life after opiates to helping

other addicts get their lives back by kicking their

addiction and personally guiding them to find the right

treatment, facilities, and aftercare. Mark makes himself

personally available to all of his readers to answer

questions and connect them to qualified professionals

and clinics. He encourages all of his readers to reach

out when they have finished the Ibogaine Journey to

find a clinic and get treatment.

Conclusion....

I have decided to write the conclusion of this book first,

a simple ending to a very intense journey. Make this a

simple reminder of the outcome you can have.

The next couple of days I was excited to just get home. I

was excited to show everyone that it was me again. I

was back, the person they knew seven years ago, and

not the lying junkie that led them down a terrible, dark,

path, my life as an addict. I had a sense of extreme

clarity, something I hadn't experienced in what seemed

like forever. I had a new sense of excitement for work,

family, and doing things I had once loved. I had needed

opiates to do anything the last seven years, because

without them I would only be sick, living in a fog, not

able to think, unable to love. I couldn't believe this

journey was ending and the outcome I had. None of it

seemed real, it truly seemed like a second lease on life.

I can imagine how an inmate serving a long sentence

must feel being released from prison. I haven't

experienced that, but feel the emotions must be similar.

You think about all the things you want to do and the

conversations you want to have with the ones you love.

You want to apologize and hug everyone that means

something to you and who had stuck with you through

the lowest of times. You want to tell the people who

decided not to support you that it was ok, you

understood, and understand why they wouldn't or

couldn't.

Ibogaine is a miracle for opiate addicts. Anyone

thinking about treatment, must learn how to

comprehend what they read online, and decipher the

half-truths and misinformation littering the Internet.

There is no other treatment option like Ibogaine, there

are no comparisons to discuss. Ibogaine is like nothing

else and the properties it has seem like they were hand-

picked to cure opiate addiction. It removes

withdrawals, crippling cravings, lack of mental clarity,

and brings back a true sense of self. It removes the

months of post-acute withdrawal symptoms that come

with typical treatment options and replaces them with

daily optimism. You can literally feel the changes in

your brain, the chemicals you were starved of flow

again, in normal proportions, balancing you. You trust

your body to be well, not needing opiates to get out of

bed. You fall in love with yourself again, something you

haven't felt since the beginning of your addiction.

If you are thinking about Ibogaine treatment, you must

take it seriously. It is powerful and must be respected.

You must be certain you have a reputable clinic, have

undergone the right medical testing, and your body is

prepared to handle the effects of Ibogaine. It can be

dangerous if you let it be. You must also be mentally

prepared. Your mind is so powerful and it must be

willing to accept the healing properties Ibogaine brings

with it. You must be willing to trust that it has curing

capabilities and accept them. You must hate your

addiction more than you love the high of the drug. You

must hate what you have done to your body, your mind,

your family. You must be willing to be cured. Love

yourself and the decision you are about to make.

Ibogaine will help you retrieve the things opiates have

stolen from you, the things you had given away to drug

addiction. Be optimistic, enthusiastic, and hopeful, and

you too can make this happen.   Best of luck, and please

feel free to reach out if you would like some guidance

and help in your journey.

Making the Decision

By the time I decided to try Ibogaine, the decision was

an easy one. Battling an opiate addiction for 7 years,

and having zero success with every treatment option

available in the United States, I was ready.

If you've been at war with your addiction for long

enough and tired of being just a junkie, you're willing to

do just about anything to say goodbye to it. Initially as I

was learning about Ibogaine and reading about the risk

factors, I started to second guess if it was the right

decision. It's difficult to say if I was having legitimate

fears about the risks of Ibogaine, or simply fears of

never using opiates again. Even with all the horrible

information I was reading online about Ibogaine,

especially the 1 and 300 mortality rate, I'm pretty

certain it was simply a fear of never using again. Addicts

are risk takers, it's just something baked in, jeopardizing

things they love and somehow rationalizing it just so

they can use. A few hair-raising statistics about

Ibogaine's risks aren't going to keep one from trying a

treatment that has a better success rate than all of the

traditional methods. If I had terminal cancer, I'd be

signed up for every experimental drug and treatment

option available, regardless of the risks.   Why would I

feel differently about my addiction? The end result

from doing nothing about it would be the same.

I will mention throughout the book brain chemistry and

how an opiate addict's brain no longer functions or

produces the proper amount of various chemicals as a

non-addict. This causes the addict to reprioritize their

emotions, how they think, and even their basic needs to

survive. They place these once important pieces of their

life and place them well behind the need to get and use

opiates. The previous example of how I was more afraid

of never using opiates again than dying during Ibogaine

treatment shows how insanity creeps into an addict and

how frustrating this could be to someone watching it

happen. That is quite profound.

Another underlying factor in my decision to try

ibogaine, something I couldn't ignore, was that

traditional treatment options for opiate addiction have

a near zero success rate. All of the rehab treatment

options cost thousands of dollars, detox you for 30 to 90

days, and send you back on the streets with massive

cravings, anxiety, depression, and reduced brain

function. None of the rehab treatment centers (that I

was aware of) addressed brain chemistry, the most

crippling aspect of the addiction's stronghold and the

reason behind the majority of relapses. An opiate

addicts brain chemistry has changed, forcing the patient

to take opiates to simply be "normal" and not

overwhelmed with anxiety, depression, reduced

cognitive function, and an inability to allow anything

important into your life, enabling personal growth. You

have no ability to feel, think, or grow when your brain is

obsessed with opiates, life comes to a standstill, simply

recycling the same 12 hours over and over again.

The alternative to rehabs, cold turkey, and tapering

methods was suboxone and methadone. Simply stated,

they are just two new opiates replacing your existing

drug of choice. I won't say that they don't have a

purpose, they do. They have saved many lives, kept

people from buying illegal drugs, and keep addicts from

ruining themselves financially. However, you are still an

opiate addict, forced into a Groundhog Day existence,

begging for your medication every 12 to 24 hours. I

tried suboxone but found myself continuing to want my

drug of choice, continuing to obsess about opiates and

never having a reprieve from addiction. It did not give

me my life back, didn't free me from my addiction, and

failed to allow me to grow as a person.

Ibogaine treatment was an easy decision at this point,

and I was ready to put all of my energy and hopes into

its success.

Once I had made my decision, my focus changed. I

concentrated on the positive information I was reading

online, watched hundreds of video testimonials of

individuals who were dumbfounded about the results,

and studied the science that was baffling physicians. I

shifted all my doubts and worry into positive energy,

simply focusing on a miracle that many others had

seemed to have had with Ibogaine. That energy shift

was important, instead of seeing a black existence in my

future, I saw hope, and couldn't wait to have it fulfilled.

I had gone through a lot to get to this point in my

addiction. I don't want to mislead folks and have them

think that all of this happened overnight. Most opiate

addicts don't use Ibogaine as their first recovery

treatment. The entire premise around the substance,

what you have to do to get the treatment, the dangers,

and the illegality, usually make it an addicts last choice.

It is unfortunate, because the success rates seem to be

much higher than traditional methods, but at the same

time, I believe the success rates would go down

significantly if it was a first-choice treatment for many

addicts. A major variable in the success of Ibogaine

depends on where an addict is within their addiction.

You need to absolutely be 100% certain, that you hate

opiates more than you love them. You are fed up with

what your life has become, the decisions you have

made, how you feel every morning, the way people look

at and judge you, the wasted years of going nowhere,

and the self-loathing weighing you down.

About 3 years prior to my treatment, I had thought I

was serious about quitting opiates for the first time. My

wife knew of my addiction, work was suffering, I was

bankrupting my family, and things seemed to be

crumbling in around me. I took the traditional route, as

most do, and entered a rehab in Pennsylvania. I was

actually confident that I would be able to quit, and I

would be one of the less than 1% who stop abusing

opiates through a traditional rehab (this success rate

varies depending on what sources you use). When

doing my research on rehab centers, I had run across

some information about Ibogaine and ended up

watching a Vice special in which they opened the

segment with "Kick the most addictive drug in the world

by using the scariest drug in the world." Not the best

way to market an addiction treatment. It didn't take

much more than that opening line, painted faces of

people hallucinating, and African tribal dances, to hit

the pause button and go back to looking at pretty

pictures of smiling families, calm lakes, and massage

therapists, curing addicts within their beautiful rehab

facilities.

My next encounter with Ibogaine was years later from

research my wife had done. By this time, she had

watched me suffer and fail countless times, witness the

ineffectiveness of every opiate addiction treatment

option, and like me, searching for a miracle to keep our

family together and her husband alive.   She sent me a

text message, it was short, and simply had a link and

one sentence that said, "Take a look at this". The

website address in the text contained the word

Ibogaine. I knew where it would lead me and decided

to ignore it. Over the course of the next couple of

weeks, I had decided to go back into pain management

in hopes to reduce the financial burden of my habit and

basically give up on quitting opiates altogether.

However, even with all of the failed attempts, I knew

deep down that if I went into pain management, I

wouldn't be swimming out of the hole I was digging for

myself. I would end up taking the prescribed dose the

doctors gave me and continue to buy off the street,

basically increasing my daily habit by 50%, not reducing

the financial burden, and driving me closer to ruining

my life and the lives of everyone around me. Pain

management would not be a solution for me, it would

simply compound my addiction and I knew it.

Instead of going to my first pain management

appointment, I reopened the text message my wife sent

and followed the link to a low budget, lousy looking,

website. I decided to look at Ibogaine with an open

mind this time. To be truthful, it really meant, I would

be looking for anything hopeful in what I read, disregard

the negative information, and justify the risks of this

treatment completely unknown to me. It is difficult to

even explain how obscure Ibogaine was (and still is).

Imagine yourself with a terminal illness, having been

diagnosed seven years prior, and spending countless

hours on the computer looking for new treatment

options, medications, and homeopathic offerings, and

finding very little. Yet with all that time and effort you

never found any consistent information about Ibogaine,

the one treatment with some of the highest success

rates and coined "nothing less than a miracle" by

thousands of former addicts. The information you

found seemed to constantly contradict itself, saying it

was very dangerous, but actually wasn't under proper

medical supervision. You would read that the clinics

were dirty and staffed with non-qualified nurses and

doctors, yet there are some who have been curing

addicts for twenty-years and have never had a death. I

am not a conspiracy theorist by any stretch of the

imagination. However, when you have an epidemic

effecting almost 10 million in the United States alone,

caused by pharmaceutical companies who downplayed

addiction rates and over prescribed painkillers, it is

difficult to ignore why information on an effective

treatment is not readily available. Your suspicions

continue as you learn more; Ibogaine is non-addictive

and has been shown to change brain chemistry. Once I

realized big pharma was not and probably won't be able

to turn a profit from Ibogaine, I was nearly convinced,

someone, was keeping it a secret, and if it weren't for

the power behind social media, no one would know of

it.

I was staying away from the Ibogaine information that

was loaded with excuses why not to use it and the

stories of death by Ibogaine and people dying during

treatment.   I instead, focused on the science, study

results, successful clinics and leaders in the medical field

who were dumbfounded by what they were seeing in

their treatment results.   Once I started looking through

a completely different perspective, changing my search

queries, and looking at the real science behind Ibogaine,

I began to see things in a much different way. I saw that

in some studies success rates were as high as 70%. For

addicts who continued to use opiates after Ibogaine

treatment, many times their usage decreased by up to

90%. But the one thing that stuck with me most, was its

ability to reduce cravings. Having gone through various

opiate treatments, I understood that the non-stop

cravings were what was keeping me and I assume many

others from succeeding. I knew that a successful

treatment program had to include changes in brain

chemistry and Ibogaine seemed to offer those

properties. Suboxone and Methadone reduce your

cravings because they are opiates. There is no other

reason, they aren't miracle drugs, they are the same

drug that you are addicted to, and when taken, reduce

cravings and withdrawals. They are both considered

successful treatment types, because they work. And to

be fair, they have saved a lot of lives. But you must be

ok with continuing to be an opiate addict, take

medication every day for the rest of your life and be

willing to deal with the long-term side effects that are

showing to be more adverse than initially indicated.

This sounds like a familiar big-pharma story, eerily

similar to what they initially claimed about Oxycontin

and Oxycodone when they hit the markets as pain

medications.

Ibogaine seemed to be different. In many of the studies

and testimonials I was reading, patients were indicating

that they had no or very little withdrawal symptoms and

cravings. This statement is so profound it sounds

impossible to any opiate addict. To simply wake up the

day after treatment and not be sick and not crave

opiates is a "to good to be true" statement. Most

addicts simply don't believe it therefore discard it as a

viable option. They halt future research simply because

they don't believe those kinds of results are feasible. It

simply sounds to good to be true. It simply can't be

possible. No way.

I decided to believe it. I decided to believe in the

people that witnessed it firsthand. I put my energy

behind the testimonials of former addicts who swear it

was a miracle. I left all my fear and suspicions about

Ibogaine behind. I had nothing else to lose at this point

in my life. I needed a reprieve from the 12-hour,

repetitive nature of my life, in which I would seek out

opiates, take them, and begin to get sick 12 hours later.

To have that cycle of insanity lifted would be a gift of life

for me.

As I dug deeper into the web's underground Ibogaine

content, other benefits that Ibogaine offered became

more consistent in the testimonials and written

descriptions of patient experiences. These benefits

included heighted senses, introspective thought, a

sense of well-being, and improved cognitive function. It

is difficult to know if Ibogaine actually improves these

things, or if removing the cycle of insanity and ingestion

of the substance allow these functions to be more

evident. Either way, if they occurred, it didn't make

much difference to me how or why it was happening.

In other parts of my story you will hear me say that I

went into treatment "blind", not knowing what to

expect, vulnerable, and unknowing about Ibogaine.

These are true statements. Although, I had done a lot

of research prior to treatment, I had nothing to

substantiate what was true, false, or half-true, so the

feeling of uncertainty, weighed on me big time. If you

read enough conflicting content, you second guess it

and tend to believe the "better looking websites" and

disregard the unknown bloggers who tended to have

the more positive experiences with Ibogaine. If you

read that Ibogaine has a 1 and 300 mortality rate, has

caused heart attacks, coma, and irreversible disabilities,

you don't ignore it, you tend to believe it regardless of

how much you have promised yourself you wouldn't

and stay focused only on the positive information. The

statements are so serious and definitive you find them

hard to disregard because of their severity. You ask

yourself, "Who would possibly write this stuff if it

wasn't true?"

Even with all of the uncertainty, the decision to go to

Ibogaine treatment was an easy one. I had tried

everything else and failed. I hated where my life was

and the inability to continue to grow. I hated being sick

every morning. I hated spending thousands of dollars

simply not to be sick. I hated the people I had to deal

with. I hated the looks on my wife and mother's faces

when they saw me. I hated being depressed and unable

to do simple tasks because of the fog my life was

drowning in. I needed help and I banked on Ibogaine to

provide it.

The Ibogaine Treatment....

I went into my Ibogaine treatment as a last-ditch effort.

I tried everything, including rehab, suboxone, tapers,

and cold-turkey. Nothing worked, and I felt nothing

would ever work. The withdrawals, cravings, anxiety,

and inability to function normally would always lead me

back to using every day. But I boarded a plane on a

Monday, in early June, out of DC to Cancun, on a

mission impossible journey, having no idea what I was

about to go through.

When I arrived in Cancun, I was high as crap, snorting

300mg of oxycodone on the flight over, mostly out of

withdrawal fear, but also as a last goodbye to the 7-year

love / hate affair I was having with prescription pain

killers.

Two young guys in a mini van picked me up. They were

dressed like nurses, almost seeming to be in disguise,

trying to look like medical professionals. They asked me

a bunch of questions about my last usage, which I lied

about, saying I was starting to withdrawal because I

hadn't used since the night before. I lied in hopes to get

more drugs, something the website had promised to

keep patients from withdrawing. Sure enough, a small

cup with a pill at the bottom was handed to me, along

with a bottle of water. I was told it was morphine and

although I had never taken it before, it sounded good at

the time.

It was about a half hour drive to the clinic which was on

the outskirts of downtown Cancun. When we arrived at

the clinic, my first impression was *wow*. It was a very

nice waterfront home, clean, with large open window's

facing the beach with a soft flow of small waves lapping

in from the Gulf of Mexico. The house was two floors,

with a lot of individual bedrooms upstairs. There were 8

or 9 individual rooms on the second floor, each with the

modern conveniences of home. All the rooms had a

wide screen TV, Netflix, major movie channels, Wi-Fi,

and a comfortable bed. To be honest, at this point I felt

a little guilty. Here I was in the tropics, away from all

my life's stress, almost enjoying myself. I mean I was

supposed to be suffering right, I was in rehab? I put on

my bathing suit and went outside and laid in the sun.

The guilt turned into a nice tan.

One of the first things I noticed was there wasn't much

going on. I didn't see many patients, or what I thought

to be patients, no group discussions or large white

boards hanging on the walls with 12 steps on them.

There were only about 7 or 8 other patients there, each

at different stages of their treatment. You could kind of

tell what treatment stage each person was in by how

they were acting. New arrivals still had the look of

uncertainly written all over their faces, patients

preparing for treatment the next day were more

reclusive, I'm sure out of fear and stress of what was to

come. The ones who just finished treatment the day

before looked sluggish, slow, weren't eating, and rarely

seen, spending most of their time in their rooms. The

folks with only a day or two left, seemed fine, almost

hopeful. I'm not saying they were taking Zumba classes

and bouncing off the walls, but they were not sick, and

most important, not dead. One consistency regardless

of how far along patients were in their treatment was

no one was overly talkative or vocal. Compared to my

other rehab experiences, where patients seemed to

socialize and form clicks, using their addictions as ice

breakers and conversation starters, the folks here were

much more isolated and reclusive. I understand why. It

is a bit terrifying, embarrassing, and their situations

probably more dire. People were not discussing their

fears, the treatment, or how they felt afterwards. If it

wasn't for my curiosity and asking others a lot of

questions, I would have known nothing about any part

of the experience. However, my intrigue had me asking

a lot of questions, trying to get a bit of insight on the

treatment and if it had worked for them.

The lack of information from both the patients and staff

was the most frustrating aspect of my experience up

until this point. I had very little to go on and felt in the

dark about what to expect. If I was to give the clinic one

critical comment, it would be they didn't properly

prepare patients with expectations. I would have

appreciated a group session in which people described

their experience and how they felt at various points in

treatment. Without that information, I became anxious.

My anxiety may have played a part in having a bad trip,

which I will describe later.

The first two days were pretty relaxed, with lots of free

time. Besides a nurse tracking me down every four

hours to take my vitals and give me morphine, I was

pretty much left on my own to do what I wanted, as

long as it was onsite. No one was allowed to leave the

property unless they were chaperoned by a staff

member and the only time that was allowed was at

11:00am each morning with a program director who

organized activities, some of which were off the

property. She organized trips to go snorkeling, visit the

local ruins, go shopping, take walks down the beach,

and attend yoga classes.

On the first day, I was scheduled for an EKG. I was told

that the EKG was the most crucial of my medical

examinations. They ran the EKG test early in your stay

because if you fail, you can't get the treatment and you

go home that day or the next. I was lucky enough to

pass. A professional hockey player was there with his

wife, both as patients, and was not permitted to go

through the treatment because of something they saw

with his heart rate. He had been denied the same day I

was being tested, so you can imagine my sense of relief

when they told me I passed and cleared me to proceed

with treatment. In the back of my mind I was thinking

there must be some serious heart concerns, but also felt

reassured that they were taking medical precautions. If

a professional athlete failed, was I going to be ok? If

you do your homework, you'll learn that many of the

medical emergencies and deaths associated with

Ibogaine treatment are heart related.

 They took me off facility on day two to get blood work

done at a local lab. It was a bit reassuring to know they

were taking such precautions. It may sound funny or

trivial, but a part of me was relieved that I was leaving

the clinic and being seen by an outside doctor at a local

business. I was still very skeptical about everything and

I thought that if something terrible happened, or I was

involved in some sort of organ extraction (a joke, kind

of) at least I was leaving a paper trail and my loved ones

could track my steps if they looked hard enough to find

my body (more jokes). Honestly, much of my skepticism

came from the lack of information from other patients

and staff members. If other patients would have been

more vocal about their experiences and the staff

conducted group sessions each night, I would have been

fine. I could have asked all my questions and hopefully

received answers that eased my mind. But having little

to no information, being alone, out of the country, and

about to take a drug that had killed people, was a bit

nerve racking. I felt the anxiety I was feeling was valid

and warranted.

Even with all of the concerns I was having, my hope

never wavered. I'll admit, there was a constant mental

battle happening within me, continuing to weigh the

concerns vs. the hope. I would remind myself that I had

done my homework, read lots of testimonials,

understood the science about Ibogaine and rationalized

why it was illegal in the United States. Even so, going to

a third world country to take a non-traditional, fringe,

psychedelic substance, that killed people, wasn't

processing well with the logical side of my brain.

I was told treatment would be on day four (of 8), so

basically it began the day following my medical

clearance. They kept me on morphine every four hours

until the day of treatment. I remember being shocked

that the 1 pill they gave me every 4 hours was enough

to keep me from getting sick. I never got a whiff of

being high from it, yet I felt fine and not craving

obsessively. I wondered what the dose was they were

giving me and I know other patients had similar feelings,

but I never did find out. It wasn't a big deal, just an

addict's curiosity. The clinic's website said you wouldn't

withdraw, but in the back of my mind, it didn't add up,

and felt I was going to feel lousy at some point, I knew

of no other way when stopping opiate use. To say I was

extremely happy I never went through withdraws is an

understatement.

As my treatment grew near, so did my curiosity. I began

asking a lot more of other patients, trying to get any

information, any insight as to what to expect and how

they were feeling post treatment.

Everyone seemed reluctant to discuss much of it in

detail. It was almost like they weren't sure if it had

worked, or it was to soon to let me know. All of them

talked about one thing though.

"THE ROOM!"

Each patient brought up "THE ROOM" when they

described their experience to me, as if it sparked some

terrible trauma they had gone through. At the time I

had no clue as to what they were talking about, or what

this room had in store for me. It wasn't until after my

treatment did it all make sense.

Looking back at everything now, it makes sense to me

why many were reluctant to open up about what they

had gone through. It is a very intense treatment and

difficult to decipher what had happened and what is

happening the first few days following treatment. You

become uncertain about your own body and experience

therefore making it difficult to open up about it to

others. It isn't like other treatments and you have

nothing to compare it to and discussing abstracts or

uncertainties isn't something most are comfortable

with. You know something is happening, and you are

very optimistic, but you certainly go through a period of

"what just happened, and am I really cured". You can't

come right out and give definitive answers as to if you

are cured or the treatment worked. However, as weird

as this is to say, you know that it didn't not work. You

aren't withdrawing, you aren't craving obsessively, and

you start to feel different. One young girl did tell me

the treatment "worked" and said she felt herself again,

but it was difficult to take her at her word, it was her

first stint in rehab, and she basically chose the one that

was only a week long, and in Cancun. So, her

testimonial validity was weak at best.

 It is one of the reasons everyone discussed the ROOM.

It was a concrete part of the experience that everyone

would be able to understand and relate to.

Since the outcome of the treatment is still up in the air

for most patients a day or two after it is administered,

patients talk about the Room they were in during the

treatment. I'll discuss this in a bit of detail later on.

Even with all of the missing information I was hoping to

have at this point, I was still hopeful and looking

forward to my treatment. I still had hope that Ibogaine,

something that many called snake oil was going to be a

miracle. I had nothing else to hope for. I was this far

along, I might as well go into it with a positive attitude.

If anything, I was curious about Ibogaine being a

psychedelic and what the trip I was about to have was

going to be like. I was looking forward to a nice

mushroom like trip, fresh with trails and vivid

hallucinations. Boy was I wrong.

The night before my treatment, I was mostly excited,

intrigued, and hopeful. I had seen and spoke with a few

others following their procedure, none were dead, none

were bed ridden, and although their description of their

experience wasn't overly satisfying to me, the fact they

were breathing and doing normal activities was enough

for me to stay hopeful.

At 8am they took me down to a small room, no

windows, just a few medical machines, a twin bed, and

a recliner chair. I was now in THE ROOM. It was

completely dark, and only enough light to get situated

and get me to my bed. I was told I would be here for 24

hours, and I started to understand what the others were

saying, the thought of being here for that long was a bit

unnerving. They put an IV in me to keep my fluids up

during the trip and EKG monitors on my chest. In what

seemed like no time at all, the doctor came in smiling

and gave me a small plastic cup. I put it in my hand,

looked down into it and saw about 6 capsules. It was

my Ibogaine.

This was my last chance to bail out. A million emotions

flooded through me. Skepticism and fear seemed to

drown out everything else. I took a moment and saw

myself just a week before crying, feeling completely

hopeless, and wishing that I could end this insanity that

had taken over my life.

It was if someone had lifted the cup to my mouth and

swallowed the pills before another thought could enter

my mind. It was as if all of my loved ones pushed that

cup to my lips and forced it into my throat, leaving me

no choice, ultimately making the decision for me.

Here we go, there was nothing to stop it now. There

was little of no hope funneling through me now. I

scanned my environment. I was in a dark room, in a

foreign country, all alone, with people I didn't know, I

was literally putting my life in their hands. I was scared, no, I was terrified. I just took a substance that I couldn't

confirm was real, and even it was, it had killed others

just like me. This moment told me a lot about what my

addiction had done to me and the risks I was willing to

take to rid of it. Yet the lengths to which I had gone

and the extreme risks I was taking somehow was worth

the small chance of defeating opiate addiction. It was a

profound moment that I decided to take a chance on.

The alternative was to go back home still an addict, get

divorced and see my kids every other weekend. I lied

my head down on the pillow. The nurse put

headphones and eye covers on me. It was to late to

turn back. I had to accept whatever outcome any

higher power and the people surrounding me had in

store.

 The music coming from the headphones was a new age

African tribal beat that repeated itself over and over. I

lied there waiting to feel something. It is difficult to

know how much time had elapsed but I began to hear a

buzzing sound, much like a helicopter, coming from a

place I couldn't figure out. On a number of occasions, I

lifted my eye cover and removed my headphones to ask

the nurse if she could hear it. She said "no" but told me

it was normal. I

started to fade into a semi-conscious state, seeing

visions, but far from what you experience with LSD or

mushrooms. It was really a sequence of thoughts, some

more vivid than others, none of it really making a lot of

sense to me. Many others who had the treatment had

said their visions were specific events of their lives

which either were directly related to their addiction or

loved ones affected by it. They describe a bit of a

storybook experience to why they became addicted,

and in many instances, the people they affected. Many

patients said this was an emotional ride, mostly

unpleasant. For me, it was more or less a lot of

different thoughts and some experiences, but nothing

connecting any dots to my addiction roots. I had

expected much more of a visual experience. Many

others had described clear visions, I was not one of

them. I felt more as if I was almost asleep (yet wide

awake at the time), similar to how you feel before you

go to bed and your mind is racing with the day's

thoughts. My emotional state was mostly indifferent, I

wasn't overly sad or happy, I was simply just

experiencing. I kind of snapped out of my trance or

dreamlike state all at once and in what seemed like only

a moment, I had become filled with anxiety. I'm not

certain what caused me to awake suddenly, but I

remember the music really started to bother me, and I

wanted it off. The repetitive sounds that were once

pleasant had become increasingly annoying. I was

mostly awake at this point and asked the nurse (who

was sitting in the reclining chair) what time it was. She

said "11:45", I had been in there less than 4 hours. The

first thing out of my mouth was "There is no way I am

staying in this room for another 20 hours", the nurse

realizing my anxiety said "you may be able to leave early

if the doctor says it is ok". Somehow this made me feel

better, thinking I would surely be let go early since I was

awake and lucid just 4 hours in to my treatment. I soon

realized I was not ok and still very much under the

influence of Ibogaine. I needed to pee, but when I tried

to get up, it was like I was extremely drunk, unable to

walk, dizzy, and blurred vision. It would have been

impossible to get to the bathroom on my own, the

nurse had to hold me up the entire walk, and didn't

leave me until I was standing over the toilet. After my

first trip to the bathroom, I lied back down and I

became extremely paranoid. A huge wave of clarity

came over me, convincing me that I had been duped,

tricked, and robbed. I played through each moment of

this journey, seeing massive holes in my optimistic

thinking, dissolving all hope that I was being cured for

my opiate addiction, rather I was being drugged and

robbed of ten thousand dollars. It all made sense, they

took my money and put me up in nice conditions so I

was happy and content the first few days. Now they

drugged me so I can't move. It all added up to a

massive scam in which they drug people into

humiliation and shame, in hopes they keep their story

to themselves.   I was convinced this was truly

happening and started to cry thinking about what I was

going to tell my wife. Wow, I had been scammed, it

seemed so obvious in that moment. Get an addict to

pay ten thousand dollars and send them alone to a

third-world country, drug them so they are

incapacitated, and when they wake up, they will be

happy to leave with their lives and nothing more.

The nurse immediately picked up on my emotional state

and asked if I was anxious. I immediately said "no, why

would I be anxious?" thinking I wouldn't let them know I

was on to the scam. She saw right through it and asked

"Mark, are you withdrawing?" I was like "What?", "Are

you withdrawing?" she asked again. I remember

reaching down and running my hands over my arms and

chest and realized I was not withdrawing, and it was at

least twelve hours since my last opiate dose. Come to

find out, it was close to twenty hours, I had been in and

out of consciousness for a few more hours and didn't

realize it. The nurse said "It's 6:00pm, it's been almost

twenty hours since your last medicine dose." I thought,

what? Twenty hours, no way. She is lying. She showed

me her phone, I read the time. Soon a sense of calm

came over me. Twenty hours without opiates was more

than enough time to make me dope sick and put me in

full withdrawals. I wasn't withdrawing. In addition, she

seemed generally concerned in how I was doing. I was

still having massive doubts about the entire thing, but at

least I was ok. I began to calm down and my anxiety

subsided slowly. The next 12 hours were brutal. I was

peeing what seemed like every few minutes, needing

help each time, still feeling drunk. I began to count the

minutes. You can't sleep, so you have to deal with hour

upon hour of lying in a dark room, second guessing

what you have done. THE ROOM was the worst! I

wanted out, now! All those promises about getting out

early were only to keep me calm, they never intended

on letting me out early, the doctor didn't even come

back to the clinic until 8am, so he couldn't approve an

early dismissal. I released on it. It didn't make the time

go any faster though. I thought, If I could only sleep, I

will wake up and be done. I knew damn well that was

not going to happen. At this point, I could feel the

stimulant properties of Ibogaine, and I wasn't going to

bed anytime soon.

They let me out of the room around 10pm to get some

air. Getting out of the room was much more important

to me than the air. The sense of confinement against

my will was lifted when I was able to leave the room.

Other people saw me come out, things seemed to be

going on as normal without me, that was reassuring to

see. I envisioned the place being empty and a group of

individuals at a table ready to tell me I had been

kidnapped and needed to follow their orders to stay

alive. It was nice to see that wasn't the case. As I sat

down outside, I soaked in the breeze coming off the

water and looked up into the full moon of the beautiful

Mexican sky. I was calmed. I was ok. I started to think

about opiates, and why I wasn't withdrawing, and why I

wasn't craving. My mind said, you aren't craving

because of the trauma you were just under, you

certainly will be in the morning.

I went back into the room in a different state. I knew I

had a few hours to go, but it was different, I was feeling

much less paranoid and was mentally preparing myself

for the remainder of the stay.

Getting out in the morning was an amazing feeling. I

was ready to go to my room and lie down, watch TV and

hopefully fall asleep. I had been up all night, but not

tired. I was up all morning and decided to go outside.

###

I made it downstairs, not to eat, I wasn't hungry, but

more out of curiosity on how I would respond to getting

around. The day before, around this time, I needed

help getting to the bathroom and was unable to stand

on my own. Just thinking about everything and how

much had happened in the last 24 hours was difficult to

comprehend. It was complete mental exhaustion. Like

I had been in a fight, one I felt I had lost, but soon would

realize I had come out on the winning end.

It was gorgeous outside, I passed a few nurses on my

way out to the pool who asked how I was doing. They

were a bit surprised that I was up and about. Most

patients spend the entire next day in bed, and

sometimes the day after. I actually felt pretty good

considering.

When I finally made it to the backdoor which led out to

the pool and the beach beyond that, I was

overwhelmed with stimulus. It was as if I was going

outside for the first time after being locked in a

windowless cell for an extended period of time. Every

sense had goosebumps, and the world was so vivid. My

sense of feeling was picking up and embracing the wind,

my eyes were saturated in colors, and I was hearing the

most minute sounds, insects, birds, the wind, the trees,

and the soft ocean waves. No one had told me I would

have these feelings. If they had, I either didn't listen, or

didn't comprehend the impact. It was almost as if I was

experiencing the "good high" from Ibogaine. The trip I

was hoping for yesterday. It was a sense of rebirth in a

lot of ways. Each step I took towards the pool was like I

was absorbing mother earth, it was remarkable.

I laid my towel down over the chair and lied down, half

reclined, so I could see out into the open bay, watching

the swaying tree tops, and the birds, perching on the

dock, fishing and watching for small breaks on the water

surface. I kept thinking I would adjust to my

surroundings, waiting for things to slowly dim to

normal. It didn't happen, just the opposite. My mind

started to open up and a smile came over me. I could

almost feel the flood of endorphins rushing through me,

spreading hope, happiness, and pleasure from head to

toe. It was as if a faucet had turned on, gushing the

chemicals I so dearly craved for the last seven years.

Chemicals that balanced me, allowed me to love, and

seek creativity, chemicals that made me who I am. The

feeling was so profound, I began to cry. I couldn't

believe it. It really happened. It couldn't be true, could

it? Was I back? I was, and it seemed better than it ever

had. I seemed improved, if that is possible. I seemed

more in tune, more conscious, more appreciative of

what i had evolved back into. I never felt I would ever

get this feeling back, get ME back in a form that didn't

need to be supplemented with opiates to survive, and

not be sick. Opiates don't make you well, although they

certainly seem like they do when you are addicted to

them. They simply keep a shell of yourself from getting

sick. You don't realize it until you get back what you

had lost. The feeling Is difficult to put words to, it was a

rebirth of some kind, a miraculous transition, that a root

from an African bush had given me. I felt so grateful. so

overwhelmed with appreciation. I wanted to shout if

from the rooftops and tell every person in the world

struggling with opiate dependency what was right here,

and it was attainable.

I was so excited to call my wife and my mother. They

had been so desperately worried about me. They had

watched their star dim each day I used, and they had

watched me fail to quit so many times, something they

were not use to seeing from me. They knew that this

drug was much more powerful and its grip much

stronger than the words you here on TV or in

magazines. This was more of something that consumed

you and nothing seemed to affect its monstrous

appetite.

For me to call and tell them what was happening, or

what had happened, would be nothing short of a

dream. Living the nightmare they had been on with me,

their son, and husband, a junkie, is truly just that, a

nightmare. I cried the entire conversation, just saying

"it worked, I'm back, I'm truly back". Not having any

idea what I had gone through, they simply knew it was

profound and real. The wave of energy and emotion

traveling 1500 miles at lightspeed from my phone to

theirs was evident and an undeniable affirmation.

This is when I knew something profound had happened.

Everything I was looking at, hearing, and feeling was

different. I was different. I felt like I had returned to a

familiar place. I soon realized that familiar place I was

feeling was my life without an addiction. It was surreal,

I was experiencing a state of being I thought I would

never feel again. I wasn't feeling a slave to opiates. My

brain had changed. I had changed. I literally went into

THE ROOM an addict and came out my former self. It

honestly was a miracle. I miracle only an addict could

understand. Looking back at everything that happened,

I believe that the initial moment you realize something

amazing has happened is an important one to your

recovery. I believe your interpretation of that moment

and how you respond to it will have a direct impact on

your success. For me it was natural, I truly was

astonished, amazed, grateful, and hopeful. I didn't let

doubts or concerns get in the way of my pure optimism.

However, I think if I would have handled that situation

with more skepticism, doubt, and disbelief, I would have

let those emotions be my self-fulfilling prophecy. I am

so glad that was not the case for me.   I remember

feeling so excited, amazed, ready to set the world on

fire. I believe this state of mind had a direct impact on

how I handled the first couple of months. I believe if I

came out of there waiting for it all to be taken away,

disbelieving what was happening, and not living in the

moment, I probably would have relapsed right away.

But my positive attitude, my appreciation of everything I

experienced, and my optimistic attitude about the

future helped frame my successful future. I was excited

to see what was next. I was excited for the experience I

was feeling.

Preparing for Ibogaine

Treatment....

What is Ibogaine?

There is a tremendous amount of information about Ibogaine online. You can learn the history, the science, uses and a lot of other good information. The real challenge is deciphering which of it is true, half-true, misleading, or false. We recommend visiting Wikipedia for general information and basic facts about Ibogaine. However, what you won't find on Wikipedia is real life testimonials and how Ibogaine is changing the lives of thousands of opiate addicts every year. To see a lot of great testimonials visit http://ibogaineclinic.com. The owner David Dardashti has been treating patients in

Mexico for nearly 20 years and has made major breakthroughs in various treatment plans for not just addiction, but PTSD, depression, diabetes, and other mental health and diseases. David in fact is the only person I know who treats opiate addicts who have been on suboxone for extended periods of time without having to switch to short acting opiates prior to treatment.

In the simplest of terms, Ibogaine is found in an African plant and is a naturally occurring psychoactive substance that has shown to drastically reduce withdrawals and cravings within opiate addicts. It's anti-addiction properties were found by mistake in 1962 by a heroin junkie named Howard Lotsof and his five friends who noted reductions of their cravings and withdrawal symptoms after taking Ibogaine as a recreational drug (it was sold in France from the 30s to the 60s as a stimulant in lower doses). Lotsof worked with a Belgian company to produce ibogaine in tablet form for clinical trials in the Netherlands and was awarded a United States patent for the product in 1985. Lotsof published his research in The American Journal of Addictions in 1999 sampling 33 heroin addicts who were given ibogaine treatment. Twenty-four of the 33 showed no signs of withdrawal or drug seeking behavior between 24 and 72 hours post treatment (typically the time period opiate addicts would be in full withdrawal). However, it should be noted that one of the 33 died, possibly involving secret use of heroin during the study, but not confirmed.

Ibogaine began to take off as a fringe heroin treatment in the early 90s with various treatment administrations being practiced, some using well developed methods and medical personnel, while others chose haphazard and possibly dangerous methodologies. In 1992 Eric Taub and Lex Kogan began to establish medically monitored ibogaine treatment clinics in several countries.

Deborah Mash, an American professor of neurology and of molecular and cellular pharmacology became fascinated with the human brain and the Food and Drug Administration of the United States granted her an Investigational New Drug license to permit her research on the addiction-stopping capabilities of ibogaine.
When a lack of funding halted her research, she began to provide assistance to Healing Transitions Institute for Addiction, a drug detoxification clinic in Cancun where physicians oversaw patients' ibogaine treatments.
Various clinics have popped up, some by Mash's trained students, who continue to provide ibogaine treatment.

Today, we have seen many ibogaine treatment clinics both come and go. However, the most reputable and safety oriented have had the most success, with one in Mexico claiming 0 deaths in 3800 treatments.

Based on ibogaine's history and results we can see that although the drug has tremendous potential in treating opiate addicts, it does have some risk, with some claiming it has a 1 in 400 mortality rate. However, with any fringe treatment, many clinics did not practice proper medical screening and monitoring, escalating the death rate, and putting a black mark on ibogaine's reputation. Finding a reputable clinic with a qualified medical staff is an important factor when choosing the right clinic for your treatment. If done right, Ibogaine is no more risky than other common surgeries or medical procedures. We highly recommend you do your research on Ibogaine and what you should be doing to mitigate risks prior to treatment.

Is Ibogaine Therapy Safe?

The following information was provided by the Global Ibogaine Therapy Alliance (http://ibogianealliance.org)

Ibogaine therapy shows a definite promise in the treatment of substance use disorder. In general, ibogaine can be administered safely and without incident, especially when done with proper preparation and supervision. However, there two interrelated issues have stood in the way of further development of ibogaine as a prescription treatment: the lack of clinical research, and the issue of safety.

Phase 1 safety trials funded by the National Institute on Health (NIH) found that ibogaine is not neurotoxic. However, because of ibogaine's systemic effects, there are certain contraindicated conditions that can pose serious health risks if not identified during a careful screening process.

Between 1990 and 2008, a total of 19 deaths were reported to be temporally associated with the ingestion of ibogaine. These incidents were attributed to a number of factors that include pre-existing cardiac conditions, seizures resulting from acute withdrawal from alcohol or benzodiazepines, and in other cases the co-administration of one or more drugs of abuse while under the influence of ibogaine.[1]

- It is crucial that patients with childhood congenital heart defects, prolong QT intervals, a history of heart failure, enlarged heart, any history of blood clots, stroke, transient ischemic attacks, pulmonary embolism, deep vein thrombosis, or irregular heart rhythms do not attempt to take ibogaine because of these risks. Other pre-existing heart conditions should be carefully examined and a risk/benefit assessment taken into consideration.
- Other conditions that should prevent someone from taking ibogaine are certain psychiatric

conditions, such as bipolar disorder, schizophrenia, depersonalization disorder, cerebellar dysfunction, epilepsy, non-substance induced psychosis, organic brain disease, and dementia. While there may be exceptions, these conditions usually do not see an improvement, and could be exacerbated by taking ibogaine.

- Impaired liver or kidney function, dehydration, and depleted electrolytes can also prevent serious risks.

- Ibogaine does not attenuate withdrawal symptoms from alcohol or benzodiazepines, and seizures, which are commonly associated with withdrawal from these substances, pose a substantial health risk. It is very important that acute alcohol detox be completed under medical supervision prior to taking ibogaine, and that benzodiazepine use be stabilized and continued throughout the treatment. Detoxification from benzodiazepines should be managed by a gradual taper after ibogaine treatment, under the supervision of a medical professional.

- One of the other causes cited in research on adverse events is ibogaine ability to potentiate the effects of opiates, as well as their lethality if co-administered. It does this not by acting as an opiate agonist or antagonist, but by enhancing opiate signaling.2 It is very important that substances are given an opportunity to fully leave the system before ibogaine is administered, and that half-lives of all substances are taken into careful consideration. This process is especially sensitive with long-acting opiates such as methadone and buprenorphine.Although many people seek out ibogaine treatment for its ability to mitigate withdrawal symptoms from short-acting opiates, it has been suggested that the safest route is to fully detox prior to ingesting ibogaine.

- In addition to attenuating withdrawal symptoms, ibogaine has been shown to reduce developed tolerance to opiates3 and alcohol,4 essentially returning the user to a novice state. Using substances after administration of ibogaine without taking this into consideration presents a significant risk of overdose.

These statistics about adverse events associated with ibogaine have been presented as a case against the development of ibogaine as a prescription medicine. However this argument does not take into consideration that those suffering from substance use disorder are a high-risk population, more than 4 times more likely to die of unnatural causes than the general population because of many of the factors associated with substance use.

Even though these statistics took into account ibogaine administration that happened in a wide variety of settings, some which included medical supervision, and many that did not, these mortality rates remain similar with those reported from methadone treatment, which is one of the most conventional treatments prescribed for opiate addiction.

In 3,414 ibogaine treatment episodes reported between 1989 and 2006, 11 resulted in a fatality. That is 1 ibogaine-related fatality per 427 treatment episodes.[6] In Australia between 2000 and 2003, 282 fatalities met the criteria for methadone-related death occurred in 102,615 TEs, which is 1 methadone-related death on 364 treatment episodes.[78] In 2004, 110 fatalities in which the medical examiner mentioned methadone as a cause of death occurred in Utah in 52,350 methadone prescriptions, which is 1 methadone-related death on 476 methadone prescriptions.[9]

It is for this reason that GITA strongly advises against the self-administration of ibogaine, and that the information presented throughout the rest of this site is considered in the context of supervised ibogaine therapy. Research supports the suggestion that professional standards for the administration of ibogaine could have a significant impact on making ibogaine therapy safer and more effective.

Are You Ready for Ibogaine?

The real truth about ibogaine is it is a miracle for many

opiate addicts who have tried everything to quit, are in

jeopardy of losing everything they love in their life, and

desperately want to get clean. Ibogaine can also be a

major disappointment for users who are not ready to

quit, don't believe in its capabilities, or have a negative

attitude about your own ability to overcome opiates.

Ibogaine is not for addicts who have major health

issues, especially heart and liver problems. You need to

get full medical screening prior to treatment and

understand the risks involved.

The Ibogaine experience will be different for everybody,

with an important variable being – *where you are in*

your addiction. If you are thinking about Ibogaine

treatment, it is essential that you are ready to quit your

addiction. You must be at a point where your hate for

the drug and the consequences it brings to your life

outweighs your love of its high. In most cases

unfortunately, this is typically a long road, and takes

time to get there. If you are being forced by loved ones

to find treatment and you are dreading getting clean or

detoxing, Ibogaine will be less effective. Like any

treatment option, the patient is the biggest factor in its

chances of success. Ibogaine treatment is no different.

If you have tried other treatment options and have

worked hard at maintaining sobriety, Ibogaine is a good

option for you. Many opiate addicts simply can't

overcome the constant cravings, the fear of

withdrawals, and the prolonged affects of post-acute

withdrawal symptoms. Many times, their lives require

them to be well and thinking clearly, which take a long

time to achieve with traditional recovery methods.

Many times patients are still not themselves after

months of sobriety, and cravings can continue for more

than a year. Chances of relapse escalate when addicts

jump back into the routines of their lives, many times

out of necessity. Ibogaine is a great option if you have

found yourself in these conditions. Ibogaine reduces

withdrawals and cravings almost immediately and

typically reduce or remove lingering post-acute

withdrawal symptoms, allowing patients to jump back

into hectic lives and schedules much faster than other

treatment options.

Finally, and probably the most important, you need to

trust Ibogaine and it's miraculous properties. Without

trust and hope of full recovery you allow negative

thoughts and feelings to take over your vulnerable state

and increase the likelihood of relapse. You will feel the

benefits of ibogaine immediately and you will be

astounded at its ability to remove obsessive cravings.

However, your ego, the one that got you addicted in the

first place, can play nasty tricks, making you feel that

you are stronger than the drug, and not at risk for falling

back into daily usage. Your ego and personality,

typically risktakers, find themselves in a similar place

after a period of being sober, in which they feel they can

handle using once in a while. Unfortunately, opiates

don't work that way, and you will be back to where you

started in a very short period of time. It is very

important to trust the properties of Ibogaine, but never

trust your ability of self-control.

Your biggest obstacle to prolonged sobriety won't be

withdrawals or cravings, it will be your own ego. Post

treatment cravings won't get you, over confidence will.

Waking up feeling normal gets you back to pre-

addiction states, but let's face it, you got there on your

own the first time, and your personality will probably

lead you directly back if you are not conscious of it, and

don't fight the thoughts of using.

My recommendation is to just go back to when you

said, "if I could only get past the withdrawals and

cravings, I would have no problems". Remember those

words, because the new you will forget them quickly. If

you are ready to face your own ego and understand that

overconfidence is probably your biggest challenge after

Ibogaine treatment, you are ready.

If you feel you are ready for Ibogaine treatment, let me help

you find a safe, reputable, facility.

The author has dedicated himself to helping others find

the right Ibogaine treatment clinics. Please feel free to

contact him at findthewaycoach@gmail.com.